child alive

by Peter Walker

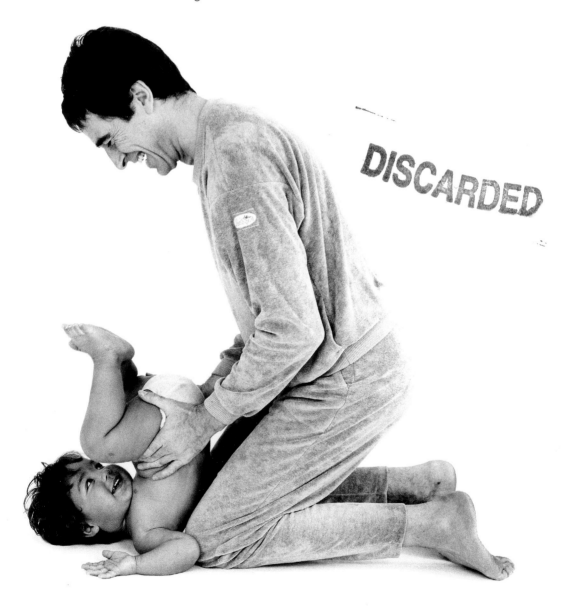

SOFT YOGA FOR INFANTS

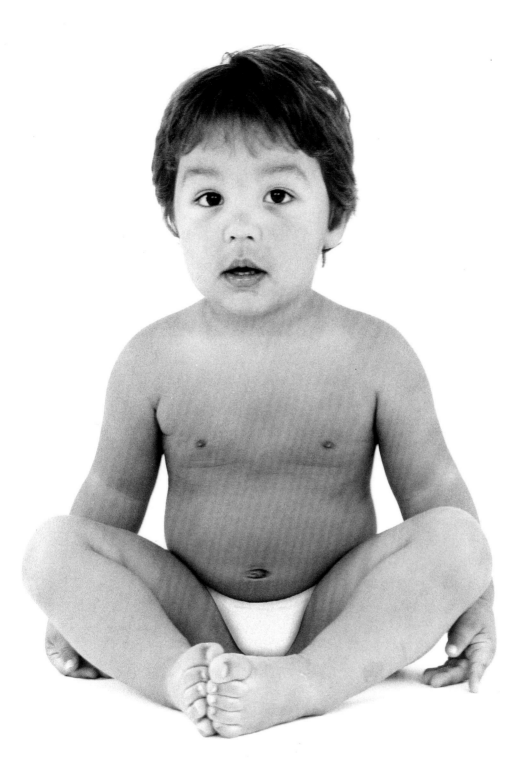

for Jason

Publishing/Text copyright
Peter Walker

Photography copyright
Dorothea Von Grief

Design & Print
Kingfisher Print and Design
Part of the ESP Colour Group

Printing History
September 2018   First Edition

Published by
thebabieswebsite.com

ISBN:
978-1-5272-2968-6

Liability disclaimer.
Check with your medical consultant
first if your child has any known
illness, disease or disability. If your
child seems unwell or resistant to all
or any of the postures. These exercises
have been safely practiced by the
author and his teachers over many
years. The author and publishers
take no responsibility for any injuries
claimed as a result of the practice of
any of these exercises.

Contents

foreword

What a world of difference this precious little book could make to children, and their parents, if taken to heart, embodied and practiced!
The loving, attentive, care-full, respectful and playful relationship we're invited and welcomed to realise with our children is here called Soft Yoga.

What Peter shows us, in his text and in the beautiful photos of him introducing his son Jason to Soft Yoga, is simply profound and profoundly simple... yet not necessarily easy.

Peter calls for a really relaxed approach on the part of the adult involved. In order to make this play work, and this work play, as well as possible, we (adults) may need to become more mindfully relaxed. What a salutary difference to our world that could make!

May you thoroughly enjoy this book and the journey it invites you to take, with love, with your children!

Dr Leon Redler MD,
Psychoanalytic Psychotherapist (UKCP registered)
Research Associate, SOAS, University of London
Honorary Consultant,
Childhood First

introduction

This beautifully illustrated book is for parents and children. It shows how to maintain a loving touch while massaging and assisting your child to enjoy some elementary stretches that will enable him or her to maintain and improve flexibility and healthy growth while strengthening the bodies muscles and joints.

Energy, flexibility and strength are the three magic ingredients of all movement. Oxygen and energy come first with a fully relaxed breathing rhythm, then flexibility enabling a wide range of versatile movement, followed by strength and coordination to restrain flexibility while securing a strong and stable body.

From birth, every child must stretch muscles to make them supple and open joints to make them flexible. These must then be strengthened to limit range of movement and establish body stability. Only movement restores, maintains and improves movement.

The simple instructions that accompany each photograph will show how best to help your child create and maintain a strong, well balanced, agile body while growing bigger and stronger.

A key concept is that everything is done in play with your child, it is not something that you impose on your child. Above all else, 'Child Alive' is fun and should be pleasurable for both parents and children. The postures illustrated may be done with your child clothed or unclothed. When massaging with or without oil, use a light touch.

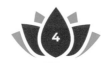

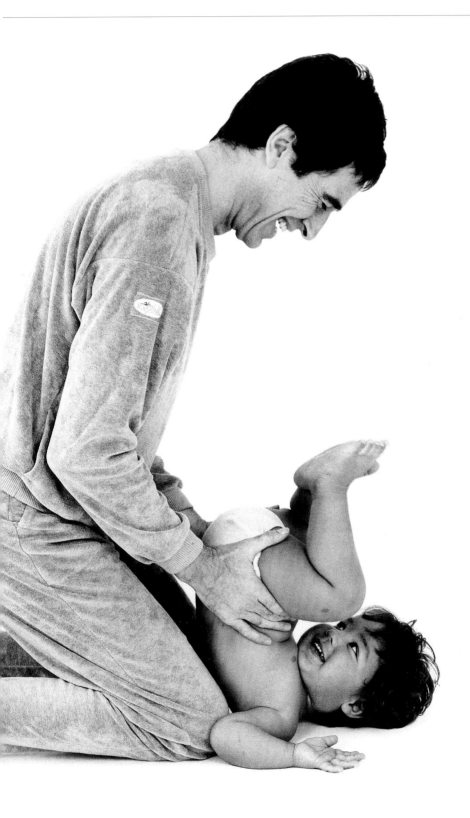

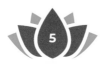

the belly

SEAT OF TRANQUILLITY

Keep the belly relaxed and you keep your child relaxed. A relaxed belly is the seat of tranquillity which allows the diaphragm to descend and maintain a deep inhalation.

It is the home of our 'gut feelings' and our 'here' and 'now' sense of reality. Breathe in for action and out to relax.

The belly influences your child 's emotional health and well-being. Emphasize the exhalation in moments of stress to remain calm and keep the body tranquil. Teach your child to 'breathe out' when stress is evident and there is a need to calm down.

Massage as shown in the illustration, distending the belly gently from side to side for a minute or two with a relaxed, cupped hand. Do not squeeze.

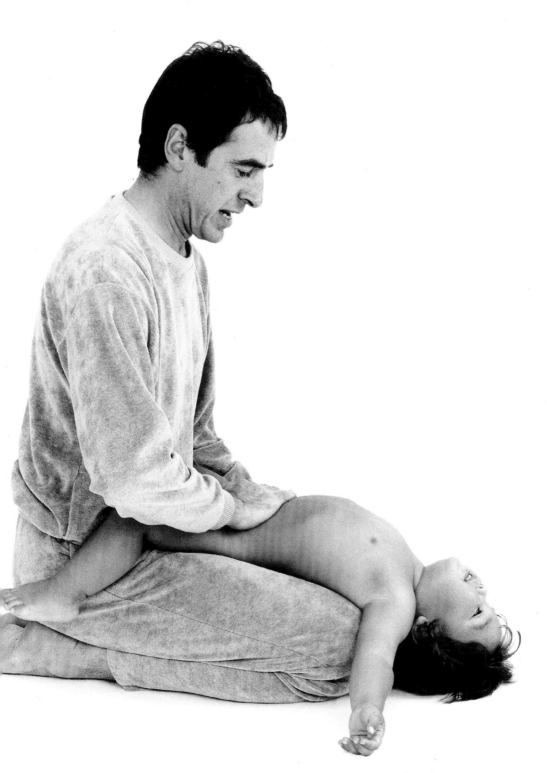

flexibility encourages a deeper breathing rhythm

the chest and shoulders

PROTECTOR OF THE HEART AND LUNGS

An open flexible chest allows for the chest and belly to work in harmony to expand and contract together. The chest should be strong enough to protect the vital organs within and flexible enough to allow a deep relaxed breathing rhythm to give all the benefits of more oxygen for less effort.

Check that your child's breathing rhythm is harmonious. This means that the belly and chest rise and fall together with every breath in and out.

Massage with relaxed open palms from the centre of the chest upwards and outwards over the shoulders and back again. Repeat this a few times.

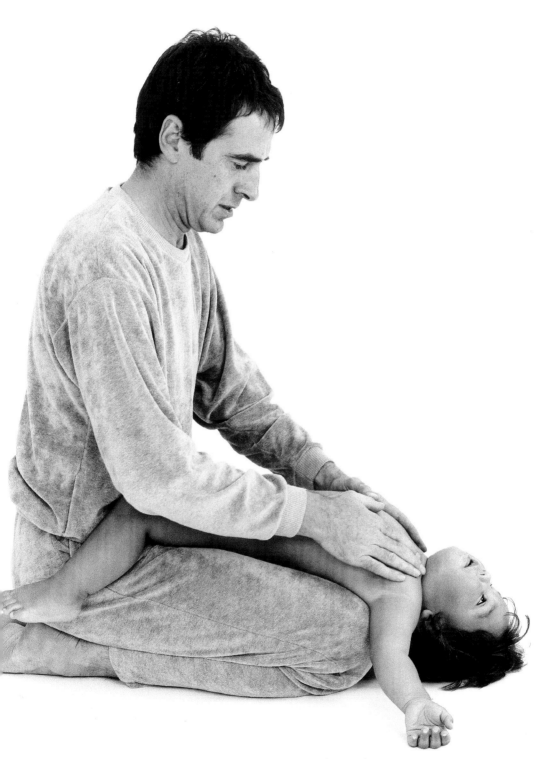

flexibility encourages relaxation

a relaxed belly and an open chest

SIGNS OF FRIENDSHIP AND WELLBEING

Oxygen is nature's nectar. Even before 'mother's milk', oxygen is our first food of life.

With every inhalation the chest expands and the diaphragm descends into a relaxed belly. With every exhalation the chest contracts and the diaphragm ascends into the lower chest.

This creates both a full and easy breathing rhythm and an internal massage, compressing and releasing the digestive organs with every breath, For infants, this takes place some 46,000 times every twenty four hours.

Keeping the front of the body relaxed and open maintains the harmony between the chest and belly.

Massage the belly, chest and shoulders with your relaxed palm, starting from the centre of the chest, down and around the navel, clockwise with light, circular movements. Repeat a few times.

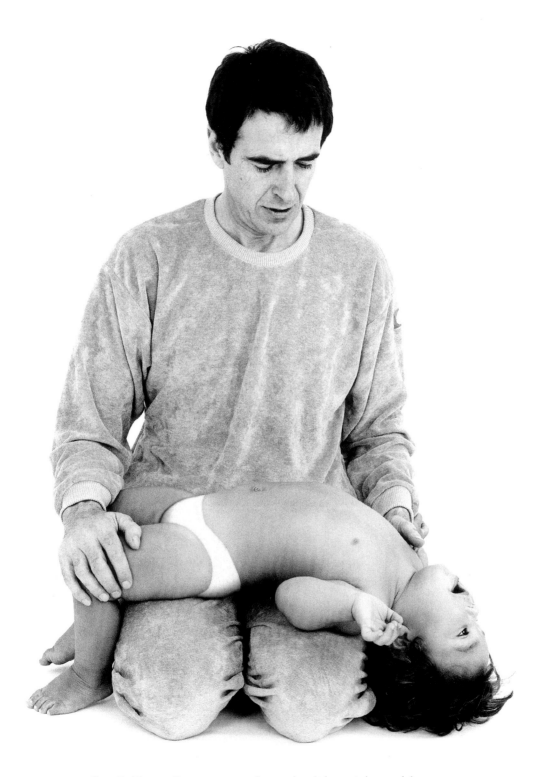

flexibility allows us to bend without breaking

the spine

A FLEXIBLE COLUMN OF FOUR EQUALLY OPPOSING CURVES

This flexible, living column of bones supports the head, the heart, the lungs and liver, arms and legs. Everything hangs off the spine and between each of its vertebrae, two root nerves emerge then divide and sub-divide to connect every living part of the body.

The integrity of this column and all that rely on it depends upon its flexibility and upon the strength and suppleness of the muscles that support it.

Stretch backwards to open the front of the body and close the back and strengthen the muscles that support the spine.

Hold securely from the hips with your knees against your child's shoulder blades, then lift your legs to enable a gentle back bend over your knees. Bring your feet to the floor to stop. Start and stop from the floor.

Hold momentarily and repeat two or three times. Keep it fun!

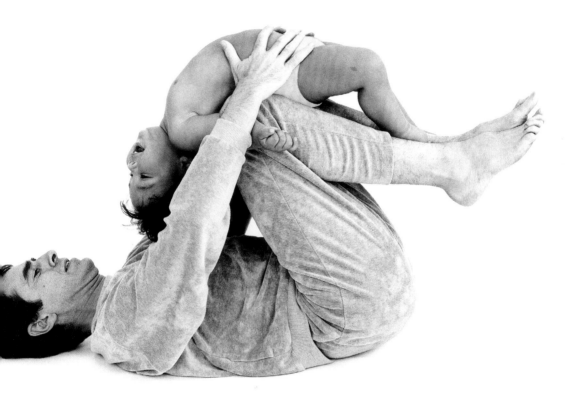

flexibility improves performance

shoulder stand

THE NECK - THE ONLY PART OF THE SPINE THAT BENDS FORWARD

To protect the vulnerable arteries and airways of your child's throat, the neck must remain relaxed to allow the chin to 'tuck in' to the breastbone. The head is balanced on the top of the spine and is supported by the strength of the upper back while the neck remains 'long' and relaxed to allow the throat to be protected

Relaxation of the neck and shoulders both protects the throat and the 'phrenic nerve' that arises from the back of the neck to control the breathing process. As this is a major nerve source to the diaphragm the flexibility of the neck and the healthy functioning of the nerve is vital to our every breath.

Support your child's body weight by a secure hold at the hips. Keeping the face forward, lift your child gently onto the back of the neck and shoulders.

Hold momentarily and while still supporting your child's weight either lift gently onto the crown of the head (see headstand - pages 16/17) or lower again gently onto the back.

Remain calm - breathe out!

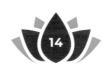

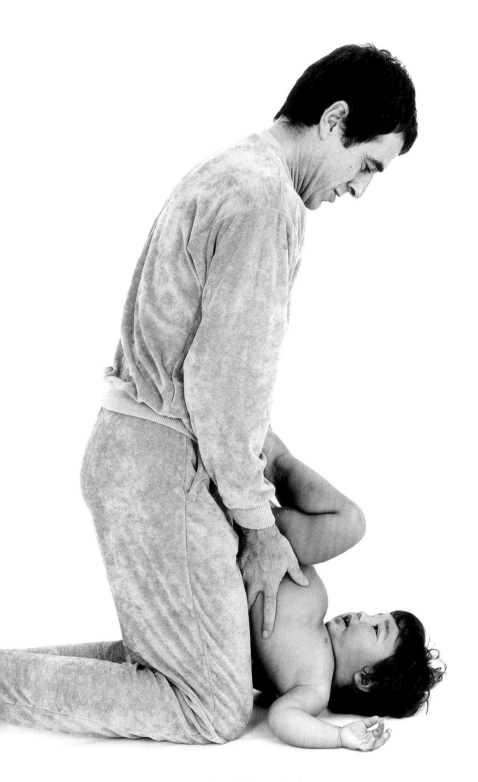

flexibility is fun

head stand

THE CROWN

There are no 'magical strings' from on high that lift us upright. Energy is the first and primal source of all movement. Our primal energy centres in the lower belly at the base of the spine from where it travels up the spine to the crown of the head.

The crown of the head is the centre from which point energy flows downwards throughout our entire body from 'top to toe'.

Meditating or focusing on the lower abdomen can raise energy levels to an extreme. This is commonly known as arousing Ki, Chi or Kundalini.

Holding your child firmly from the hips lift onto the crown of the head and supporting your child's full weight, hold momentarily before lowering gently and slowly downwards onto the back. Keep it fun!

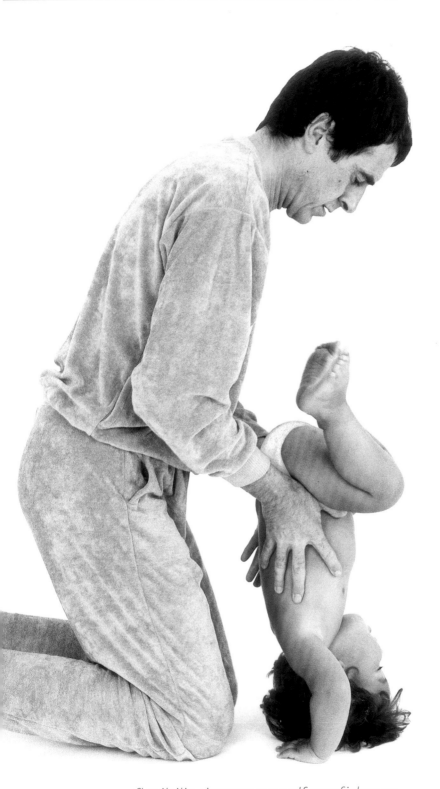

flexibility improves self confidence

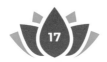

handstand

ARMS AND SHOULDERS

Standing upright gives us free use of our arms and hands, a huge turning point in human evolution. Free movement of the arms, hands and shoulders, is essential to our work and daily life and our sports and games.

One of the recreations best loved by children and adults alike is swimming, an activity that demands the free movement of the arms and shoulders.

For the ancient Greeks swimming was a highly prized accomplishment equivalent to intellectual learning. It was said of those uneducated that 'they neither new their letters nor how to swim'.

A simple handstand can maintain the free movement of the arms and shoulders. When pushing upwards while being held in this position, it extends the wrists and the hands and coordinates, stretches and strengthens the arms and stabilises the shoulders.

Lift and support your child's weight securely in a handstand by holding from the lower legs above the ankles. Encourage your child to push with their hands. Hold momentarily before lowering gently downwards onto the back.

Keep it relaxed, keep it fun.

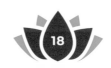

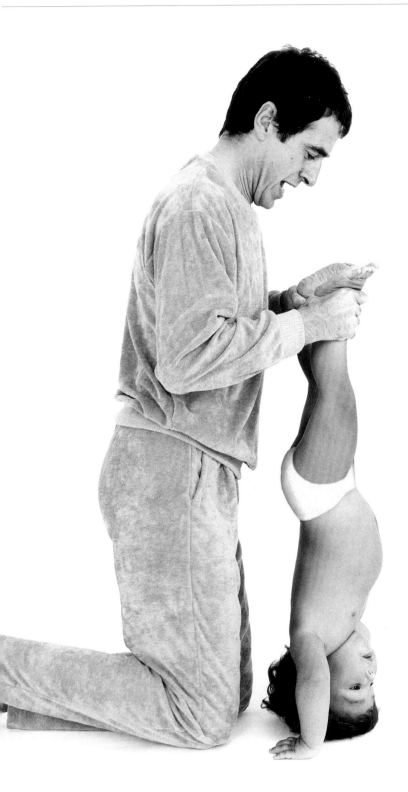

flexibility encourages good muscle tone

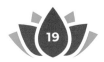

hand stand to back bend

THE SACRED SPINE

The spine is also known as Jacob's Ladder and the Stairway to the Stars. The strength and coordination of the supporting muscles and the flexibility of the spines joints allows this living column of thirty-three interlocking bones to flex, extend and twist. But of all the movements enabled by the spine none is greater than its ability to bend back on itself.

The body's joints are organs of movement. If their range of movement is inhibited then their function is inhibited. If their function is inhibited they cannot be said to be healthy. Flexibility of the spine is implicit in good health.

The first part of the movement illustrated in the photograph opens the chest and shoulders and strengthens the arms, shoulders and upper back.

From a prone position on the floor assist your child to lift into handstand and then supporting the lower back securely, let the back bend and the legs drop slowly towards the floor, first stretching and opening the chest and shoulders.

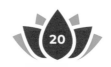

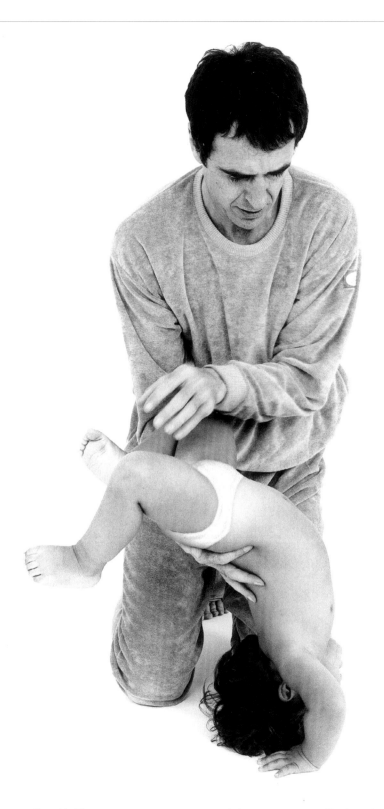

flexibility encourages a wider range of physical activities

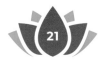

back bend

A FLEXIBLE SPINE NEEDS STRONG SUPPORTING MUSCLES

The spinal column is the first living structure that forms inside the womb. It is from the spine that the human body and its limbs take root. The flexibility of the spine is crucial to balanced posture and ease of movement.

Ancient physicians equated good health with 'A good bodily feeling' in which flexibility was an important feature. Flexibility and the art of gymnastics is thought to have evolved from Aesculapius who achieved such fame as a physician he was said to be the son of Apollo, the Greek god of health.

From the handstand to backbend illustrated in the previous exercise, support the lower back and chest, and let the belly and front thighs stretch and the feet touch the floor.

While still fully supporting the spine, as the toes touch the floor follow through and assist your child onto their feet and up into a standing position.

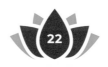

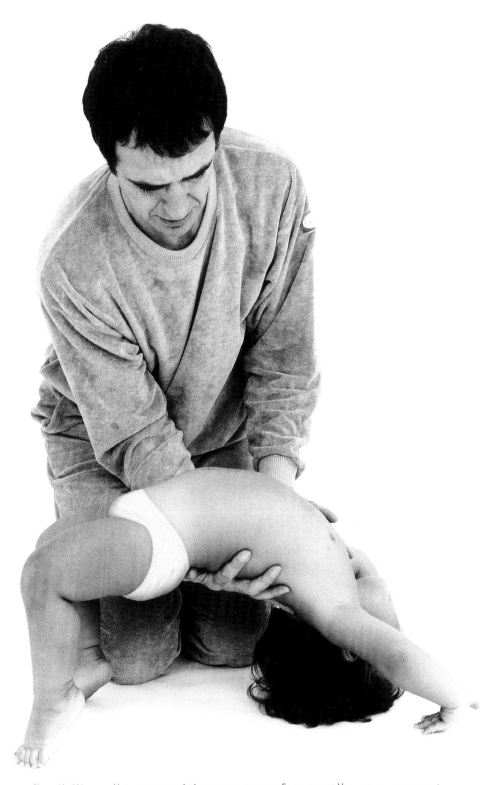

flexibility allows a wider range of versatile movement

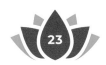

twist

THE SPINE ROTATES

During the 'Golden Age' of Greece, a time from which great myths and legends and the Olympic games evolved athletes were advised 'not to develop one physical attribute at the expense of another'.

In physical development flexibility precedes strength.

Rotation of the spine is an integral part of an agile body. The spine twists and rotates from side to side through the upper back and this exercise maintains the rotation of the spinal column while opening the shoulders and releasing the lower back.

Place one hand lightly on the shoulder of your child as the other hand gently rotates the hip and leg in the opposite direction.

Hold momentarily, rock gently and repeat for both sides. Relax and keep it fun!

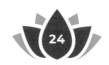

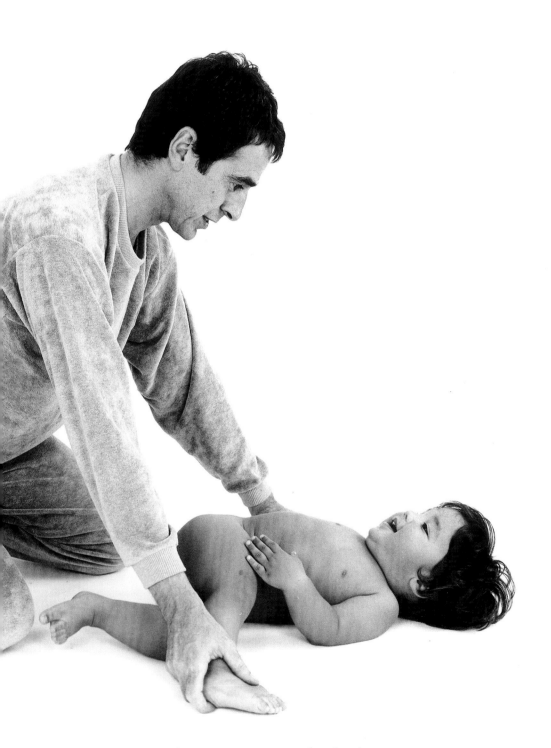

flexibility encourages physical ease

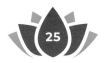

the legs

THE ROOTS OF STABILITY

Hippocrates, a famous Greek physician, known as 'the father of modern medicine' made flexibility synonymous with good health around 500 BC. He was the first to record a system of gymnastic exercise in 'Corpus Hippocraticum' which from that time on held a recognised place in therapeutic medicine.

Muscles are organs of power and sensation. Their suppleness is essential to feelings of ease and the mobility of the joints and limbs that they serve.

The legs are the body's roots pushing down from the hips to ground the body. The hips allow forward bending of the trunk. The knees, as the largest and lowest single weight bearing joints of the body, bear the most weight. The ankles are a structural masterpiece that cushion the body's entire weight to literally 'put a spring' into our every step.

Bending forward from the hip stretches and releases the calf muscles and hamstrings. As demonstrated in the photograph, gently assist your child to bend forward, then hold momentarily, Gently pat your child's back. Keep it fun!

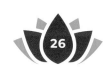

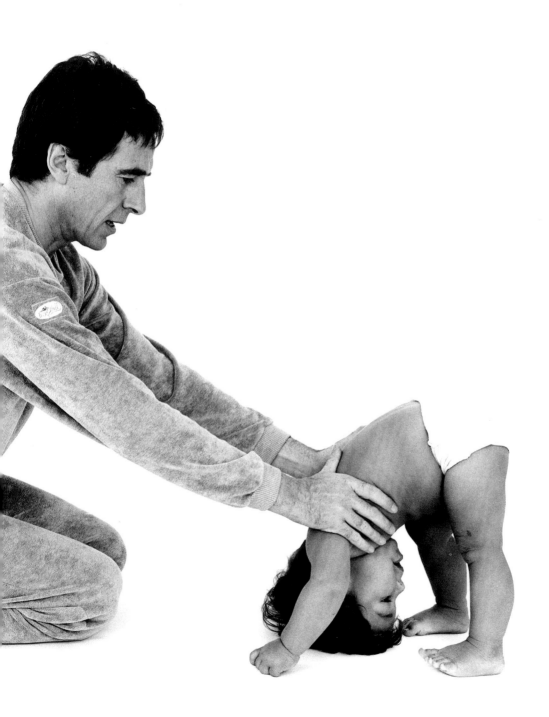

flexibility feels good

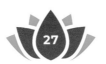

the legs

ENABLE MOBILITY

Following the Ancient Greeks, during the Roman Empire Galen was the most popular physician, equating flexibility with health. He claimed that 'gymnasts are the masters of exercises of youth with an understanding of their strength and power'. As such, 'gymnasts instruct athletes and all others in what has medical bearing'.

Sitting on the back of the thighs in front of the buttock bones maintains the flexibility of the hip joints and the integrity of the spine. Mobility demands the hip, knee and ankle joints be flexible.

Starting with our ankles our balanced bodies in motion depend upon the health of these joints.

In this exercise, pull the buttocks out so your child is sitting in front of the buttock bones on the back of the thighs. This allows the spine to bend freely forward from the hip joints. Hold momentarily.

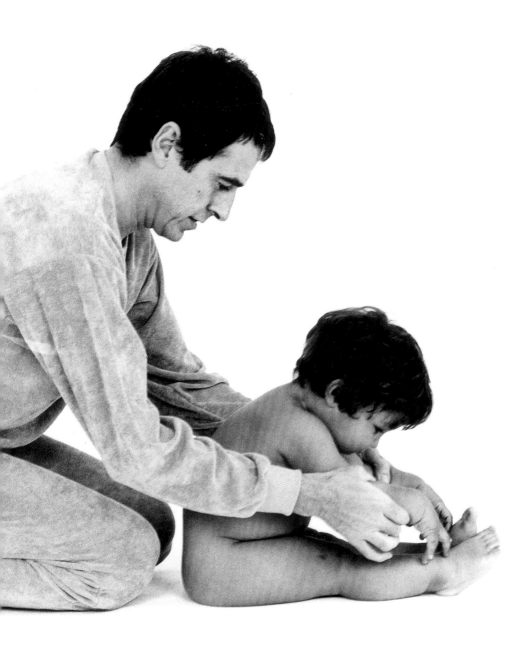

flexibility reduces the chances of physical injury

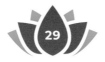

the legs

ENABLE ELEVATION

The renowned Arabian physician Avicenna promoted flexibility. In a tenth century medical text he recorded gymnastic movements which remained in use in the universities of Lourain and Montpellier up to the eighteenth century.

Standing, walking or running, our legs lift, balance, support and move our entire body weight. Supple muscles and flexible joints equate with physical ease in posture and mobility because the body's weight remains centred through the joints.

Leaning forward in the position shown in the photographs keeps the hip joints flexible and enables the spine to remain straight and 'free' when bending forward while both sitting or standing.

Gently massage the back with your palms for a minute or two to help relax your child in this position and encourage good posture. Stay relaxed and keep it fun!

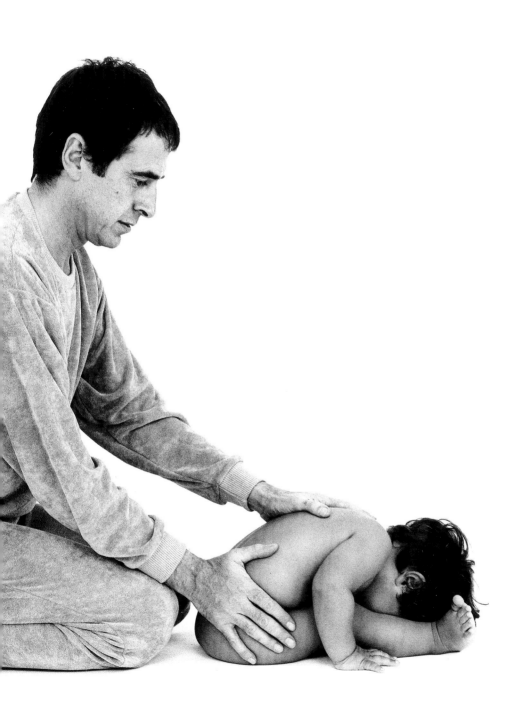

flexibility reduces the effects of physical injury

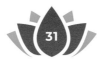

the legs

PROVIDE PHYSICAL SECURITY

During the sixteenth century educationalists again promoted flexibility alongside physical health and creative attainments claiming 'those well versed in gymnastic exercise were far more likely to accomplish the immense achievements associated with the great exertions of ancient Greek and early Renaissance artists'.

The exercise illustrated here allows for more physical contact but has essentially the same benefits as the previous exercise. It will keep the hip joints flexible and enable the spine to remain straight when bending forward, both in standing and in sitting.

Sit comfortably and hold the legs from above the ankles. With both knees turned outwards rock the feet towards the face.

Hold momentarily and rock gently from side to side.

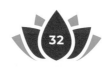

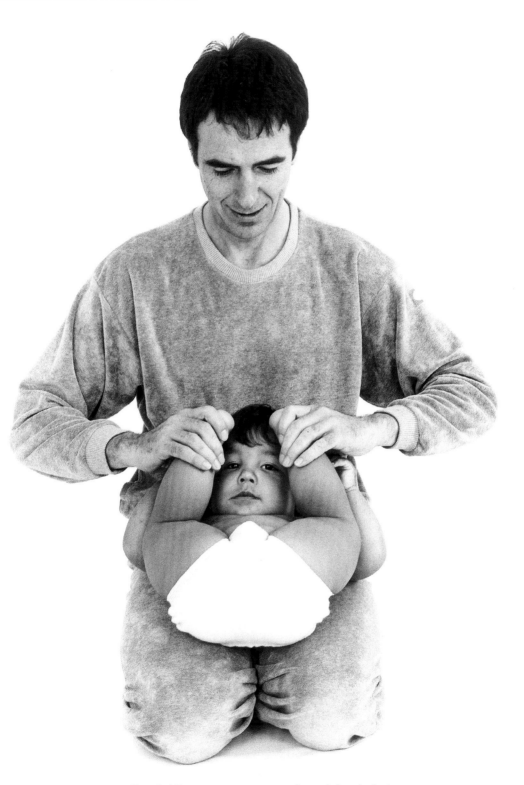

flexibility encourages healthy joints

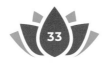

the legs

GROUND THE BODY WHEN SITTING

During the sixteenth century Heronymus Mercurialis, a university teacher and physician, wrote and promoted 'De Arte Gymnastica' in which he argued that 'the physical education of our youth deeply influences the public health of our culture'.

Following on from the previous exercise, allow the legs and knees to bend gently outwards stretching the inside thighs.

Sit comfortably and holding the legs from above the ankles and with both knees turned outwards, rock gently from side to side. Hold momentarily.

These muscles tighten quickly to keep the legs together once your child becomes upright and mobile, and their suppleness is important to the flexibility of the hip joints and the free movement of the legs.

The flexibility of the joints and suppleness of the muscles is of equal importance to our circulation and the nerve impulses that span and connect throughout our body.

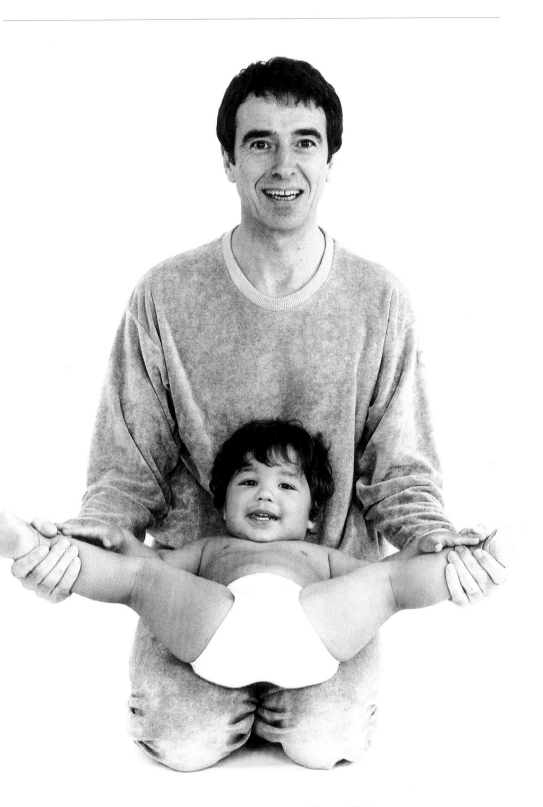

flexibility encourages self confidence

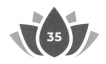

the legs

GROUND THE BODY WHEN STANDING

Flexibility and agility exercises were introduced into nineteenth century education throughout Europe by Pehr Henrik Ling and Frederick Ludwig Jahn. The exercises were accepted into the educational systems of Sweden, Germany, Denmark, Russia and America.

A regimen of free form exercise to promote flexibility and agility was practiced daily by children in schools throughout the UK until the 1960's.

Another fun way of doing the exercise already illustrated, is to let the legs open and the knees bend outwards, as shown here. Hold from the feet and rock gently side to side.

Supple postural muscles promote the health and flexibility of the supporting joints.

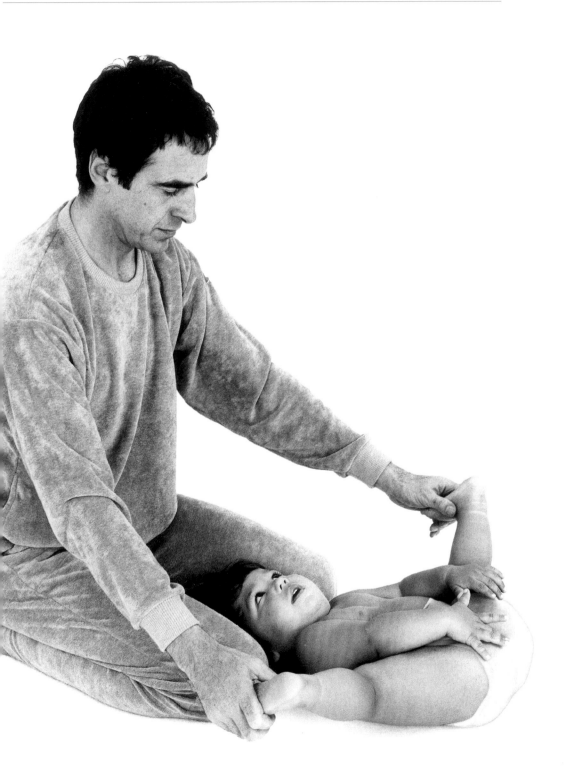

flexibility accompanies healthy muscles

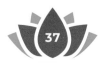

the legs

ENABLE A BROAD BASE FOR BALANCE

During infancy as children grow and their bodies develop they become little weight lifters through daily lifting and carrying their rapidly increasing body weight.

To make balance easier when first standing, these inside thigh muscles remain relaxed to allow a wide stance and a broader base for balance. Once walking and running, in order to keep the legs together, these muscles begin to tighten.

These stretches will maintain suppleness as these powerful muscles strengthen. As flexibility must precede strength, introducing these fun therapeutic stretches will enable your child to strengthen and retain a wide range of versatile movement.

While sitting behind your child, ensure that he or she is sitting on the back of the thighs in the illustrated position.

With the palms of your relaxed hands, stroke over the top of the thighs and knees to the ankles. Repeat several times.

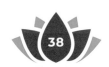

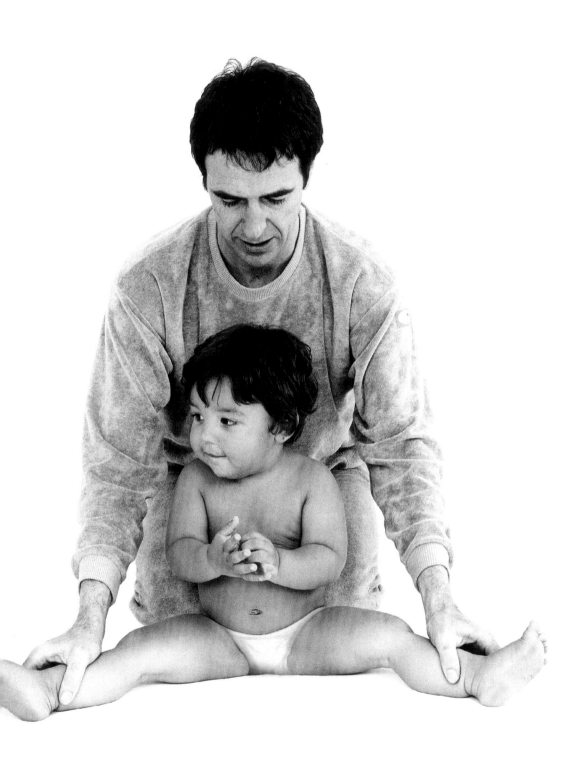

flexibility accompanies muscular suppleness

the legs

ENABLE THE VENOUS RETURN

The body depends upon its roots for mobility and security. One of the most highly prized Olympic events for the ancient Greeks was running, as this was deemed the sign of a free man.

Flexibility and suppleness is especially important in the legs as their movements stimulate the 'venous return'; that is, the return circulation of blood to the heart against the force of gravity.

For this exercise, maintain the position previously illustrated and encourage forward movement to stretch the inside thighs and hamstrings and keep hip joints flexible. This allows a broader base and the spine to remain free while bending forward.

Massage lightly, stroking downwards and outwards from the upper back down over the top of the thighs and knees, using the relaxed palms of your hands.

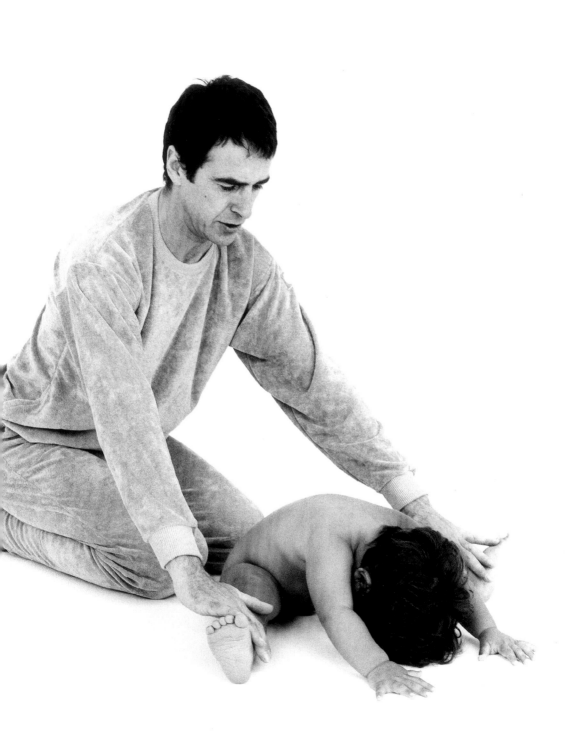

flexibility and agility go together

forward bend to first sitting position

PREPARES FOR FIRST SITTING POSTURE

Feet together with the knees open is the first sitting position in nature's motor milestones. This posture demands flexible knees and hips to enable a broad base to sit on, which makes balancing easier.

The photograph illustrates a sitting position that encourages the flexibility of the hips and knees in one leg while stretching the back thigh and calf muscles of the other leg. Practicing this will make it easier for the child to rest on the back of the thighs and sit up straight in first sitting.

With your child leaning forward in this position stroke down the back with the palm of a relaxed hand. Repeat for both sides of the body.

Making it fun while helping your child to do this will help to maintain ease and flexibility in what is known as the 'tailor pose' – your child's first sitting position. This is a posture that will last a lifetime.

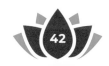

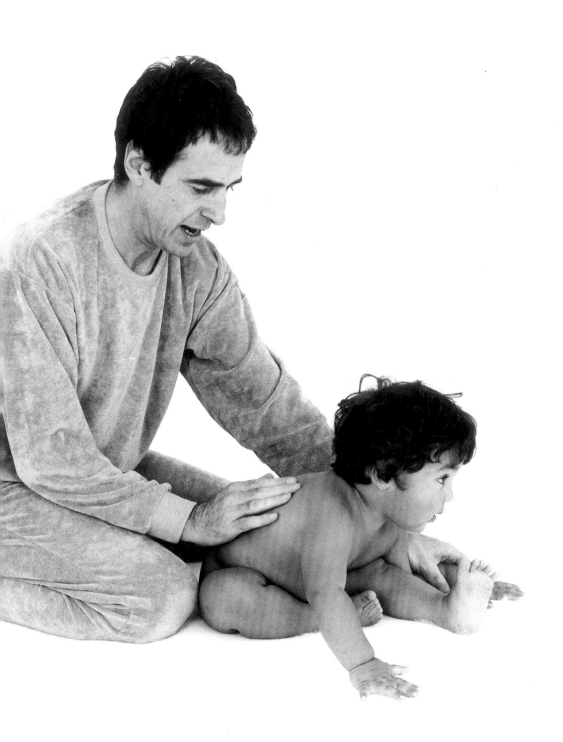

flexibility encourages a pain free body

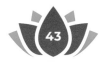

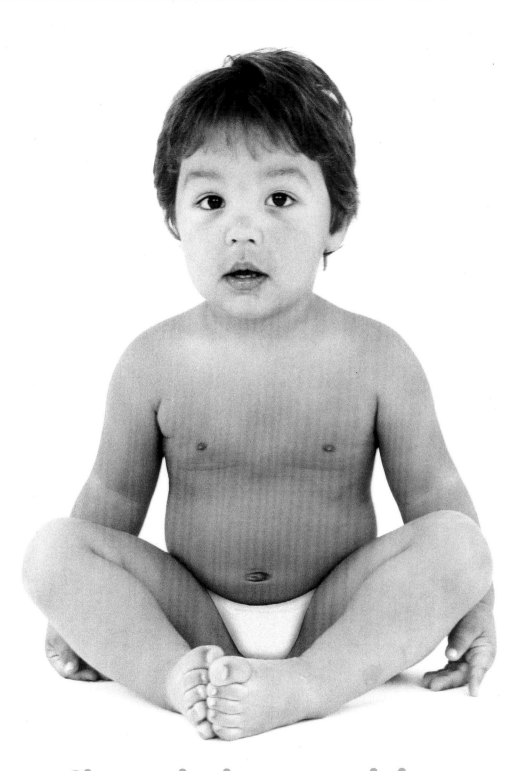

first sitting position

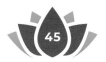

first sitting position

SITTING ON THE LEGS

The broad base needed to assume this position requires supple inside and back thigh muscles and flexible hips and knees. Being well grounded down through the legs releases the spine the arms, hands and shoulders and makes balanced movement easier.

Good feelings of strength and self-confidence come from being well grounded. Whether standing or sitting, feeling the support of gravity holding us from below is of great emotional significance. It is something that most of us take for granted.

Sit behind your child in the position shown and rest the palms of your relaxed hands over the inside thighs, close to the groin. Press down gently to open the legs from the hips to provide a broad stable base to sit on.

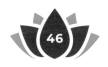

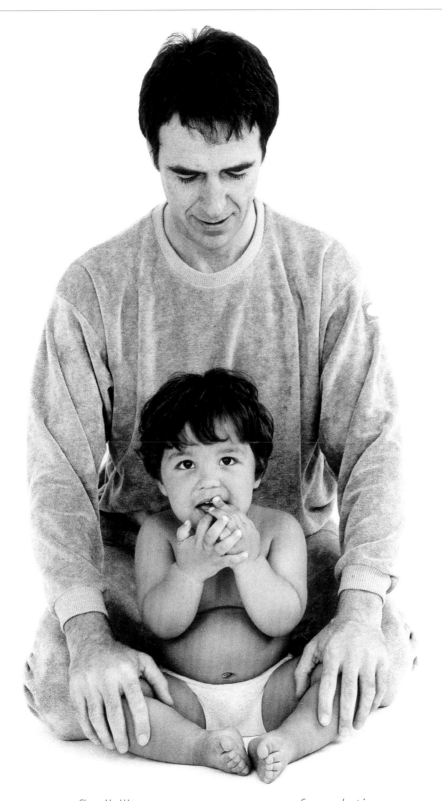

flexibility encourages secure foundations

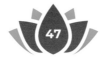

first sitting position

LAYING FORWARD

Sit up straight, from leaning forward in this position, you will feel the flow of energy divide as the base of the spine and the legs push down and the spine lifts up and straightens. Sitting and standing with strong roots encourages a secure well-balanced posture.

This position stretches the inside thigh muscles, flexes the knees and ankles. This encourages the child to sit on the back of the legs while keeping the hips and the knees flexible.

The first sitting position is most often used in meditation to raise our primal energy. Traditional yoga texts claim that sitting focused in this way rejuvenates the body.

With your child sitting on the back of the thighs encourage bending forward. This movement frees the spine and as the energy flows upwards it enables the spine to lift and extend. Use relaxed palms to stroke gently hand over hand down your child's back.

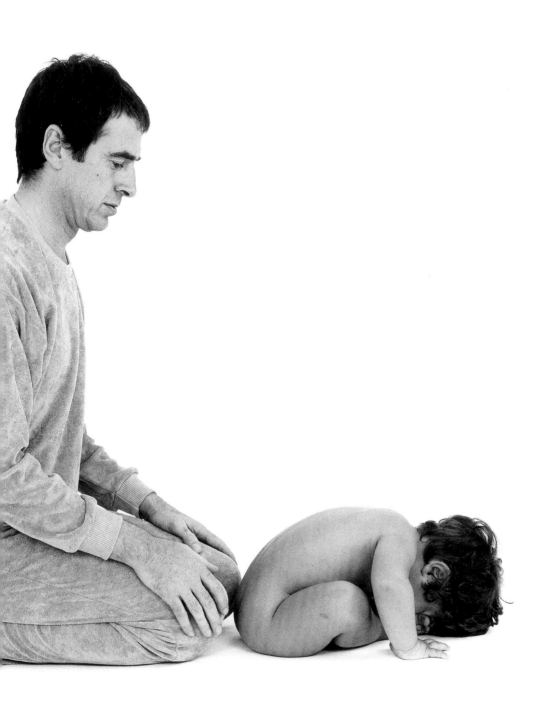

flexibility frees the spine

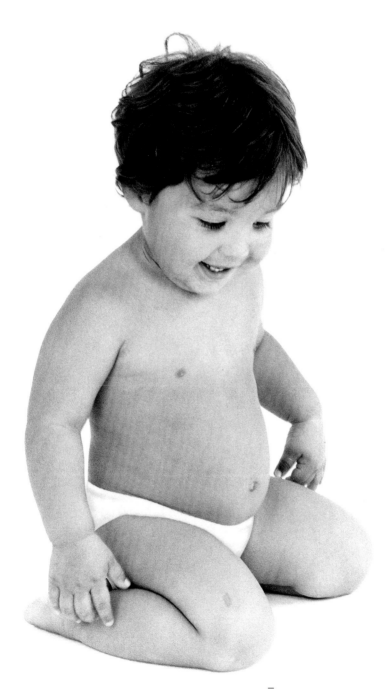

second
sitting position

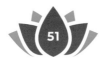

second sitting position

SITTING ON THE FEET

The second sitting position allows the spine to remain straight and bend forward with more ease. The second sitting position flexes the knees and extends the ankles, this will keep both the knees and the ankles flexible. In this position leaning forward comes more easily from the hip joints.

The ankles are an architectural masterpiece. A series of beautifully sprung arches that cushion the body with every step. The upright body relies on their flexibility to remain balanced in motion.

Once sitting on the legs and feet the ankles and toes must turn inwards. This retains the integrity of the ankles and prevents hyper mobility of the knees and hip dislocations.

Take Note: Turning the feet outwards (sitting in a W position) can damage the hips and knees and render the ankles stiff.

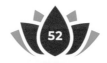

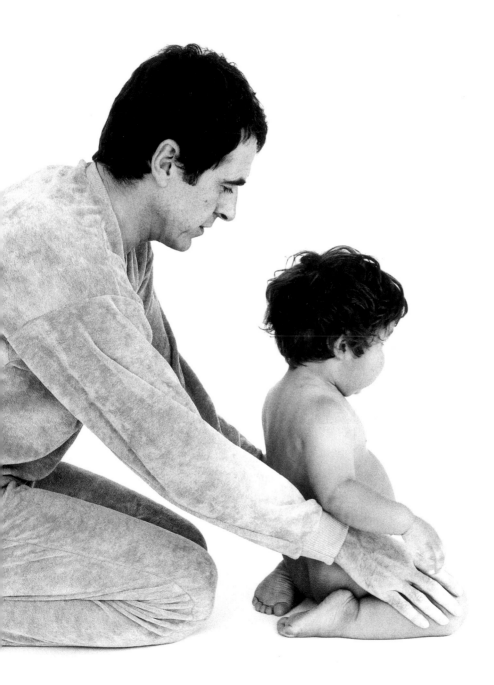

flexibility encourages well balanced posture

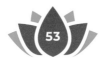

second sitting position

LAYING BACK

The front of the thigh consists of four powerful muscles known as the quadriceps. Part of their function is to bend the knee and lift the leg. These muscles are generally tense following birth as the knees are kept tucked into the trunk during the last months of confinement.

They often take a little time to relax and release the 'physiological flexion' that this imposes. Missing 'tummy time' can leave these powerful muscles tighter for a longer period of time.

Leaning back in this position stretches and relaxes the front thighs which in turn will help straighten and strengthen the lower back when upright.

Let your child lean back over your knees and thighs. Gently rub the front of the thighs with the relaxed open palms of your hands.

Breathe out and keep it fun!

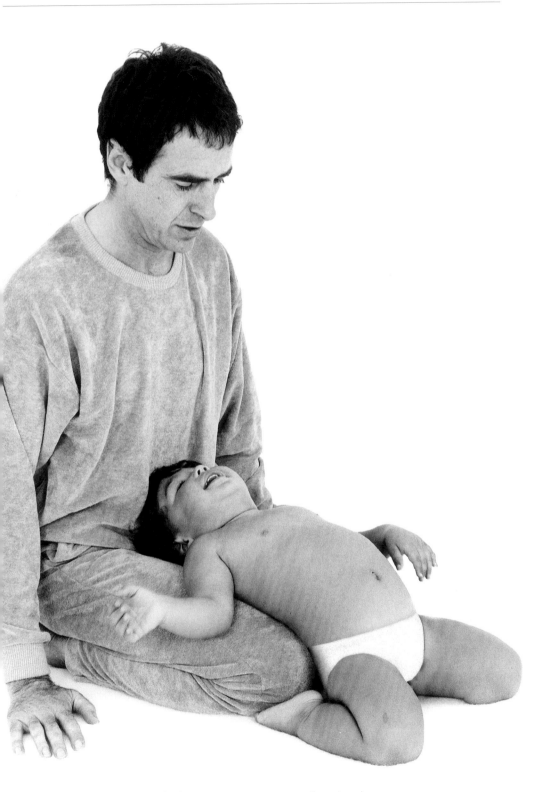

flexibility encourages physical ease

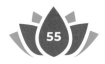

third sitting position

SQUATTING

In order to stand up-right from first or second sitting position the child must first 'squat'. Squatting is nature's way of making the legs stable before your child stands up-right and is a regular sitting position in many parts of the world.

Sitting to standing comes in three stages.

Stage one, squatting brings the knees over the feet and causes the lower legs to push down to spread the feet and toes and anchor the heels down.

As the child begins to lift from this position he or she must then lean forward into stage two and push down through the whole leg from the hips only then can the spine engage, stage three, and lift the trunk into an up-right position.

Rock the knees gently over the feet three or four times to stabilize the lower legs, ankles toes and heels in squatting, before standing upright.

Keep it fun. Make this a game

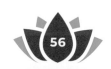

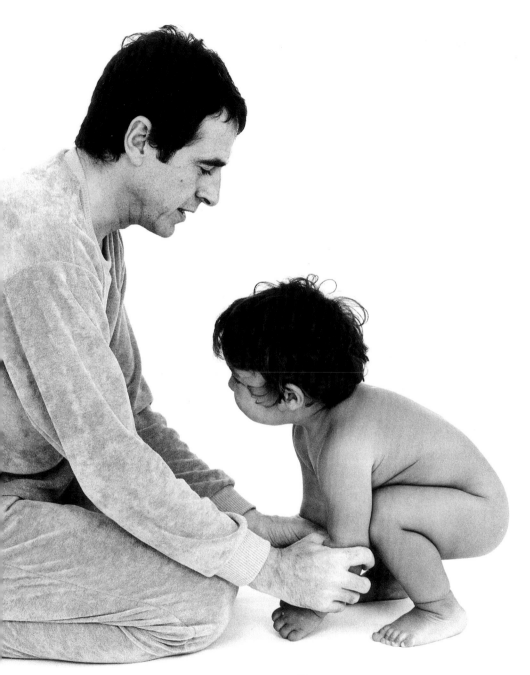

squatting

flexibility and stretching go together

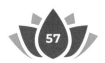

squatting to crawling

CRAWLING LINKS THE DEVELOPMENT OF THE BRAIN WITH THE BODY

Now crawling, for the first time the child is able to gain the independence to move away from you rather than you moving away from him or her.

Crawling stimulates the left and right hemispheres of the brain and as the brain simultaneously processes hearing, sight and mobility, the more a baby crawls the more these skills synchronize and develop..

Crawling is something that extends later to intellectual learning as it stimulates different areas of the brain that are of importance to future learning.

Crawling stimulates body/brain development through repetitive movement, and develops cognitive processes such as concentration, memory and comprehension.

Crawling stabilises the hands, arms and shoulders and presents the opportunity to learn and discover spatial concepts like under, over, in and out

Crawling is an important stage in motor development. Encourage lots of crawling activities. Enjoy crawling races, hide and seek, crawling from room to room and other crawling games and activities that can be made fun!

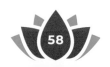

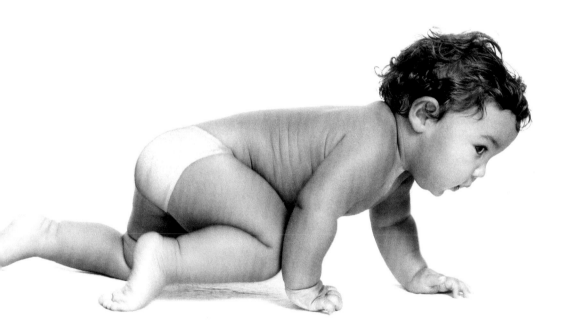

crawling

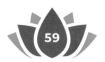

standing

REACH FOR THE MOON

This is a lovely little stretch to keep the front of the body open and the back strong. Do not pull your child from their hands or wrists. The child's wrists are one of the last parts of the body to develop. It takes some years before all the bones of the wrists are complete.

Hold from the forearms above the wrists and let your child lean back against your thighs to lift up on their toes. This will help your child stand straight with their shoulders set back and down in a gravity friendly stance.

When the head, neck and shoulders start to 'droop' gravity begins to pull the body forward. As the back starts to round it loses its strength. This playful stretch can assist your child to maintain a well balanced posture. Hold momentarily and continue to next position.

Keep it fun!

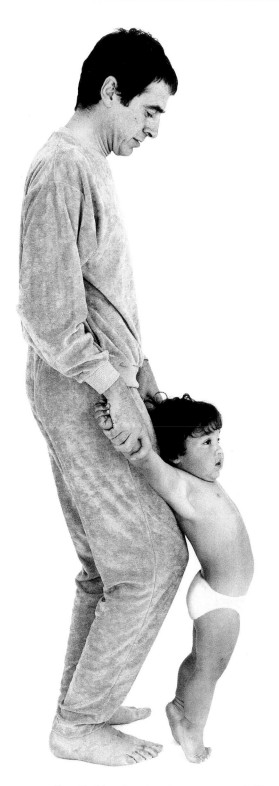

flexibility is the key to stability

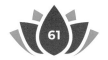

standing

STRETCH TO THE STARS

Continuing on from the previous stretch, while still holding the forearms from above the wrists with your child still leaning back against your thighs let both feet drop to the floor.

Stretch gently to open the arms and shoulders while rocking from side to side a couple of times before slowly releasing.

Maintaining well balanced up-right postures allows the front of the chest to open and the shoulders to 'set back'. This position allows gravity to pull the body up instead of over.

This helps to conserve energy and keep the back 'pain free'.

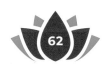

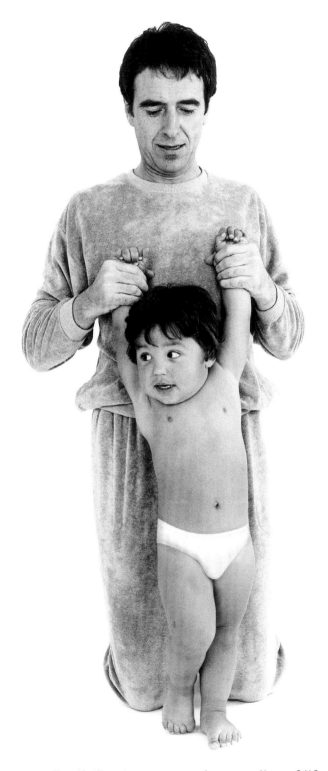

flexibility improves the quality of life

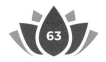